OVERCOMING MULTIPLE SCLEROSIS DIET COOKBOOK FOR SENIORS

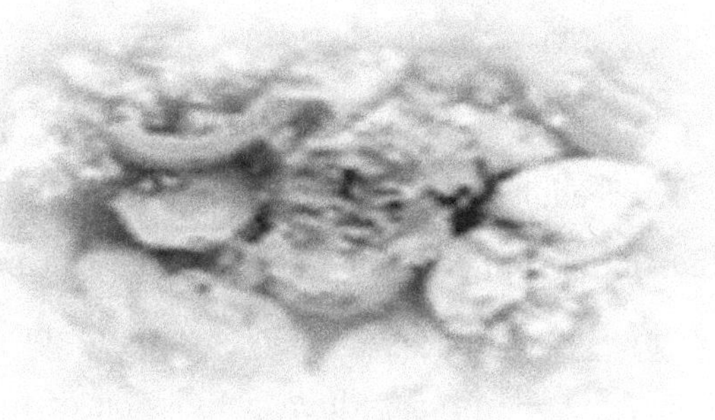

Quick and Easy Anti-Inflammatory Recipes, Low Fat diet and Meal Plan to Manage MS Disease.

David T. Salcedo

Table of Contents

INTRODUCTION

My experience with MS started with a diagnosis that hit me like a ton of bricks. I was having a great career and a wonderful family life when I began to have weird symptoms in my mid-30s. I was weak, tired, and unsteady on my feet. My struggle through testing, appointments with doctors, and uncertainties finally resulted in the diagnosis of multiple sclerosis, which changed my life.

Having Multiple Sclerosis was a struggle. Because the illness was so unexpected, organizing even the most basic activities was difficult. I frequently experienced chronic weariness, trouble moving around, and mental fog. While some symptoms were alleviated by conventional therapies, the side effects were becoming more and more problematic. I was committed to finding a non-pharmaceutical means of enhancing my quality of life.

I first learned about the importance of diet when I began looking into alternate methods of treating MS. It has been suggested by a number of studies and anecdotal evidence that dietary modifications may have a beneficial effect on MS symptoms. Motivated by these tales of optimism and recovery, I made the conscious choice to take control of my health by implementing a diet that prioritized whole foods and particular nutritional guidelines.

I started my change by gradually switching to a diet that focused on the essential elements listed below:

- Anti-Inflammatory meals: To lessen inflammation in my body, which is frequently the cause of MS symptoms, I included meals high in antioxidants, like fruits and vegetables.

- Omega-3 Fatty Acids: Eating walnuts, flaxseeds, and fatty fish helped lower inflammation and promote brain function.

- Elimination of Trigger Foods: I determined which foods made me feel better and cut them out of my diet. This includes dairy, gluten, and processed foods, as some MS patients may have increased inflammation as a result of them.

- Gut Health: A balanced immune system and general well-being were promoted by a focus on gut health through the consumption of foods high in probiotics and prebiotics.

I started to see noticeable improvements in my health as I stuck to my new diet plan. My mobility improved, and the chronic lethargy that had been plaguing me began to subside. I also felt more invigorated and had improved mental clarity. I was able to lessen my dependency on drugs over time, which improved my wellbeing even more.

Using diets to help me overcome multiple sclerosis was a very life-changing experience. Although I am aware that not everyone can be cured by food alone, it has been extremely helpful in both managing my MS symptoms and enhancing my quality of life. By means of meticulous investigation, trial and error, and the counsel of medical experts, I discovered a route towards enhanced health and overall wellness. My experience is a living example of the transformative power of diet and what happens when we take charge of our own health.

What is Multiple Sclerosis

The central nervous system, which includes the brain and spinal cord, is impacted by the autoimmune disease known as multiple sclerosis (MS), which is chronic and frequently debilitating. Myelin, the layer that protects nerve fibers, is wrongly attacked by the immune system in multiple sclerosis. The normal passage of electrical impulses along the nerves is disrupted by this attack, which causes inflammation, damage, and the formation of scar tissue (sclerosis) on the myelin. Consequently, a wide range of symptoms, varying in severity, can be experienced by people with MS. These symptoms may include fatigue, muscle weakness, difficulty with balance and coordination, vision impairments, and cognitive impairment.

Types of Multiple sclerosis

- This form of Multiple Sclerosis is called and it's the most common form of it.. Relapses, or worsening of symptoms, are experienced by people with RRMS, which are then followed by remissions, or partial or full recovery.

- Secondary-Progressive MS (SPMS): A small percentage of people with RRMS eventually develop SPMS, which is distinguished by a more consistent course of the illness with or without sporadic relapses.

- Primary-Progressive MS (PPMS): This less prevalent kind of MS is characterized by a progressive deterioration of symptoms from the start and lacks a clear pattern of relapse and remission.

- Relapsing MS (PRMS): This is the rarest kind, in which patients have acute relapses interspersed with a stable course of the illness.

Causes of Multiple Sclerosis

Although the precise etiology of multiple sclerosis is still unknown, environmental and genetic factors are thought to play a role. Among the theories are:

- Dysfunction of the Immune System: Multiple Sclerosis (MS) is believed to be an autoimmune illness in which the myelin sheath that surrounds nerve fibers is mistakenly attacked by the immune system.

- Genetics: Although MS is not inherited directly, there is a genetic component because the condition tends to run in families. Susceptibility may be increased by specific genes.

- Environmental Factors: MS may develop as a result of exposure to specific viruses, infections, and vitamin D insufficiency, among other things.

Symptoms of Multiple Sclerosis

A wide range of symptoms, varying in intensity and duration, can be produced by multiple sclerosis. Typical symptoms consist of:

1. weariness: One of the most prevalent symptoms is severe, persistent weariness.

2. Weakness in the Muscles: Decreased strength and lack of coordination might impact movement.

3. Numbness or Tingling: Individuals with multiple sclerosis frequently report having numbness or tingling in different body areas.

4. Vision Issues: Damage to the optic nerve may result in double vision, blurred vision, or pain in the eyes.

5. Problems with Balance and Coordination: Imbalance and poor coordination can cause issues with walking and other daily tasks.

6. Cognitive Changes: Memory, focus, and problem-solving skills can all be impacted by MS.

7. Bladder and intestinal Dysfunction: Urinary or intestinal issues can affect some people.

Prevention of Multiple Sclerosis

While there is presently no way to prevent MS, there are certain techniques that may assist manage its symptoms or lower the risk of having the disease:

1. Vitamin D: Sufficient levels of vitamin D may help lower the incidence of MS. Dietary supplements and sun exposure both have advantages.

2. Healthy Lifestyle: Adopting a non-smoking lifestyle, eating a balanced diet, and exercising frequently will improve general health and perhaps lower the risk of MS.

3. Early Diagnosis and therapy: Appropriate diagnosis and prompt therapy can help control symptoms and impede the disease's advancement.

4. Medication: A number of disease-modifying treatments (DMTs) are available to control the symptoms of multiple sclerosis (MS) and lower the incidence of relapses.

5. Stress Management: Stress-reduction methods like yoga and meditation can assist people in managing the mental and physical difficulties associated with multiple sclerosis.

CHAPTER 1

Breakfast Recipes

1. Berry and Greek Yogurt Parfait

Ingredients

- 1 cup Greek yogurt

- 1/2 cup mixed berries (strawberries, blueberries, raspberries)

- 1 tablespoon honey

- 1/4 cup granola

Preparation

- Layer Greek yogurt, mixed berries, honey, and granola in a bowl.

- Repeat the layers as desired.

- Serve immediately.

Nutritional Information

- Calories: 350

- Protein: 15g

- Carbohydrates: 45g

- Fat: 13g

- Fiber: 5g

Serving Size: 1 parfait

Preparation Time: 5 minutes

2. Avocado and Spinach Breakfast Wrap

Ingredients

- 1 whole wheat tortilla

- 1/2 avocado, mashed

- 1 cup baby spinach

- 2 eggs, scrambled

- Salt and pepper to taste

Preparation

- Spread mashed avocado on the tortilla.

- Add baby spinach and scrambled eggs.

- Season with salt and pepper.

- Roll up the tortilla and serve.

Nutritional Information

- Calories: 350

- Protein: 15g

- Carbohydrates: 30g

- Fat: 18g

- Fiber: 8g

Serving Size: 1 wrap

Preparation Time: 10 minutes

3. Oatmeal with Almonds and Banana

Ingredients

- 1/2 cup rolled oats

- 1 cup almond milk

- 1/4 cup sliced almonds

- 1 ripe banana, sliced

- 1 tablespoon honey (optional)

Preparation

- Oats should be cooked with almond mink by following the instruction on the package.

- Top with sliced almonds, banana, and a drizzle of honey if desired.

Nutritional Information

- Calories: 400

- Protein: 10g

- Carbohydrates: 50g

- Fat: 18g

- Fiber: 8g

Serving Size: 1 bowl

Preparation Time: 10 minutes

4. Vegetable and Goat Cheese Omelet

Ingredients

- 2 eggs

- 1/4 cup chopped bell peppers

- 1/4 cup diced tomatoes

- 2 tablespoons crumbled goat cheese

- Salt and pepper to taste

Preparation

- Eggs should be whisked in a bowl then add salt and pepper.

- Heat a non-stick pan, add eggs, and cook until set.

- Add bell peppers, tomatoes, and goat cheese.

- Fold the omelet in half and serve.

Nutritional Information

- Calories: 320

- Protein: 15g

- Carbohydrates: 6g

- Fat: 25g

- Fiber: 2g

Serving Size: 1 omelet

Preparation Time: 15 minutes

5. Smoothie Bowl with Spinach and Berries

Ingredients

- 1 cup spinach

- 1/2 cup mixed berries (strawberries, blueberries, raspberries)

- 1/2 banana

- 1/2 cup almond milk

- 2 tablespoons chia seeds

- 1/4 cup granola

- Sliced almonds (optional)

Preparation

- Blend spinach, mixed berries, banana, and almond milk until smooth.

- Pour the smoothie into a bowl.

- Top with chia seeds, granola, and sliced almonds.

Nutritional Information

- Calories: 350

- Protein: 8g

- Carbohydrates: 50g

- Fat: 15g

- Fiber: 12g

Serving Size: 1 bowl

Preparation Time: 5 minutes

6. Quinoa Breakfast Bowl

Ingredients

- 1/2 cup cooked quinoa

- 1/4 cup plain Greek yogurt

- 1/4 cup diced apples

- 2 tablespoons chopped walnuts

- 1 tablespoon honey

- Cinnamon (optional)

Preparation

- In a bowl, layer quinoa, Greek yogurt, diced apples, and chopped walnuts.

- You can sprinkle with honey and cinnamon, if desired.

Nutritional Information

- Calories: 330

- Protein: 10g

- Carbohydrates: 45g

- Fat: 12g

- Fiber: 5g

Serving Size: 1 bowl

Preparation Time: 10 minutes

7. Chia Seed Pudding with Mango

Ingredients

- 3 tablespoons chia seeds

- 1 cup almond milk

- 1/2 cup diced mango

- 1/4 teaspoon vanilla extract

- 1 tablespoon shredded coconut (optional)

Preparation

- In a jar, mix chia seeds, almond milk, and vanilla extract.

- Leave overnight inside the refrigerator or for few hours until it thickens.

- Top with diced mango and shredded coconut before serving.

Nutritional Information

- Calories: 280

- Protein: 7g

- Carbohydrates: 30g

- Fat: 15g

- Fiber: 11g

Serving Size: 1 serving

Preparation Time: 5 minutes (plus refrigeration time)

8. Buckwheat Pancakes

Ingredients

- 1/2 cup buckwheat flour

- 1/2 cup almond milk

- 1 egg

- 1/2 teaspoon baking powder

- 1/2 teaspoon cinnamon

- Sliced bananas (optional)

Preparation

- In a bowl, whisk buckwheat flour, almond milk, egg, baking powder, and cinnamon until smooth.

- Heat a non-stick pan and pour the batter to make pancakes.

- Serve with sliced bananas if desired.

Nutritional Information

- Calories: 290

- Protein: 9g

- Carbohydrates: 40g

- Fat: 10g

- Fiber: 6g

Serving Size: 2 pancakes

Preparation Time: 15 minutes

9. Rice Cake with Almond Butter and Berries

Ingredients

- 2 rice cakes

- 2 tablespoons almond butter

- 1/2 cup mixed berries (strawberries, blueberries, raspberries)

Preparation

- Spread almond butter on rice cakes.

- Top with mixed berries and serve.

Nutritional Information

- Calories: 300

- Protein: 7g

- Carbohydrates: 40g

- Fat: 14g

- Fiber: 6g

Serving Size: 2 rice cakes

Preparation Time: 5 minutes

10. Sautéed Spinach and Mushroom Scramble

Ingredients

- 2 eggs

- 1 cup fresh spinach

- 1/2 cup sliced mushrooms

- 1/4 cup diced onion

- Salt and pepper to taste

Preparation

- Sauté mushrooms and onions in a pan until softened.

- Add spinach and cook until wilted.

- Whisk eggs in a bowl, then pour them into the pan.

- Cook until set, season with salt and pepper, and serve.

Nutritional Information

- Calories: 280

- Protein: 15g

- Carbohydrates: 10g

- Fat: 20g

- Fiber: 3g

- Serving Size: 1 scramble

- Preparation Time: 15 minutes

CHAPTER 2

Lunch Recipes

1. Grilled Chicken and Quinoa Salad

Ingredients

- 4 oz grilled chicken breast

- 1/2 cup cooked quinoa

- 1 cup mixed greens

- 1/4 cup cherry tomatoes

- 1/4 cup cucumber slices

- Balsamic vinaigrette dressing

Preparation

- Grill the chicken until cooked through.

- Assemble the salad by combining mixed greens, quinoa, cherry tomatoes, and cucumber.

- Top with grilled chicken and drizzle with balsamic vinaigrette.

Nutritional Information

- Calories: 350

- Protein: 30g

- Carbohydrates: 30g

- Fat: 12g

- Fiber: 5g

Serving Size: 1 salad

Preparation Time: 20 minutes

2. Lentil and Vegetable Soup

Ingredients

- Dried green or brown lentils of 1 Cup

- 4 cups vegetable broth

- 1 cup diced carrots

- 1 cup diced celery

- 1 cup diced onions

- 2 cloves garlic, minced

- 1 teaspoon cumin

- Salt and pepper to taste

Preparation

- Rinse lentils and combine with vegetable broth in a pot.

- Add vegetables, garlic, and spices.

- Simmer for 20-30 minutes until lentils and vegetables are tender.

Nutritional Information

- Calories: 300

- Protein: 18g

- Carbohydrates: 55g

- Fat: 2g

- Fiber: 18g

Serving Size: 1 bowl

Preparation Time: 40 minutes

3. Spinach and Feta Stuffed Chicken Breast

Ingredients

- 4 oz chicken breast

- 1 cup fresh spinach

- 2 tablespoons crumbled feta cheese

- 1 teaspoon olive oil

- Salt and pepper to taste

Preparation

- Preheat the oven to 375°F (190°C).

- Cut a pocket into the chicken breast and stuff with spinach and feta.

- Season with salt and pepper.

- Heat olive oil in an oven-safe pan, sear the chicken, then bake for 20-25 minutes.

Nutritional Information

- Calories: 320

- Protein: 40g

- Carbohydrates: 3g

- Fat: 16g

- Fiber: 2g

Serving Size: 1 chicken breast

Preparation Time: 30 minutes

4. Salmon and Quinoa Bowl

Ingredients

- 4 oz grilled or baked salmon

- 1/2 cup cooked quinoa

- 1/2 cup steamed broccoli

- 1/4 cup diced red bell peppers

- Lemon-dill sauce (made with Greek yogurt)

Preparation

- Cook the salmon as desired.

- Assemble the bowl with quinoa, salmon, steamed broccoli, and bell peppers.

- Drizzle with lemon-dill sauce.

Nutritional Information

- Calories: 350

- Protein: 30g

- Carbohydrates: 30g

- Fat: 12g

- Fiber: 5g

Serving Size: 1 bowl

Preparation Time: 25 minutes

5. Quinoa and Black Bean Salad

Ingredients

- 1 cup cooked quinoa

- Black beans (canned, drained and rinsed) of 1 Cup

- 1/2 cup diced red onion

- Diced bell peppers (red, yellow, or green) of 1/2 cup

- 1/4 cup chopped fresh cilantro

- Lime vinaigrette dressing

Preparation

- In a large bowl, combine quinoa, black beans, red onion, bell peppers, and cilantro.

- It should be Drizzled with lime vinaigrette dressing and toss to combine.

Nutritional Information

- Calories: 320

- Protein: 12g

- Carbohydrates: 55g

- Fat: 4g

- Fiber: 12g

Serving Size: 1 salad

Preparation Time: 20 minutes

6. Chickpea and Spinach Salad

Ingredients

- Canned chickpeas, drained and rinsed of 1 Cup

- 2 cups fresh spinach

- 1/4 cup diced red onion

- 1/4 cup cherry tomatoes

- Lemon-tahini dressing

Preparation

- In a bowl, combine chickpeas, fresh spinach, red onion, and cherry tomatoes.

- Sprinkle with lemon-tahini dressing and toss to combine.

Nutritional Information

- Calories: 340

- Protein: 14g

- Carbohydrates: 45g

- Fat: 14g

- Fiber: 10g

Serving Size: 1 salad

Preparation Time: 15 minutes

7. Black Bean Salsa with Baked Sweet Potato

Ingredients

- 1 medium sweet potato

- 1/2 cup black bean salsa (canned or homemade)

- 2 tablespoons plain Greek yogurt

- Fresh cilantro for garnish

Preparation

- Bake the sweet potato until tender.

- Split it open and top with black bean salsa.

- Garnish with Greek yogurt and fresh cilantro.

Nutritional Information

- Calories: 330

- Protein: 10g

- Carbohydrates: 70g

- Fat: 1g

- Fiber: 15g

Serving Size: 1 sweet potato

Preparation Time: 45 minutes (baking time)

8. Tuna and White Bean Salad

Ingredients

- 1 can (5 oz) tuna, drained

- Canned white beans, drained and rinsed of 1 Cup

- 1/4 cup diced red onion

- 1/4 cup diced celery

- Lemon-tarragon dressing

Preparation

- In a bowl, combine tuna, white beans, red onion, and celery.

- Drizzle with lemon-tarragon dressing and mix well.

Nutritional Information

- Calories: 320

- Protein: 30g

- Carbohydrates: 35g

- Fat: 5g

- Fiber: 10g

Serving Size: 1 salad

Preparation Time: 10 minutes

9. Eggplant and Tomato Stew

Ingredients

- 1 medium eggplant, diced

- 1 can (14 oz) diced tomatoes

- 1/4 cup diced bell peppers

- 1/4 cup diced onions

- 1 clove garlic, minced

- Olive oil

- Italian seasoning blend

Preparation

- Heat olive oil in a pot and sauté onions, bell peppers, and garlic until soft.

- Add eggplant, diced tomatoes, and Italian seasoning.

- Simmer until the eggplant is tender.

Nutritional Information

- Calories: 280

- Protein: 6g

- Carbohydrates: 50g

- Fat: 8g

- Fiber: 16g

Serving Size: 1 bowl

Preparation Time: 30 minutes

CHAPTER 3

Dinner Recipes

1. Baked Salmon with Asparagus and Quinoa

Ingredients

- 6 oz salmon fillet

- 1 cup asparagus spears

- 1/2 cup cooked quinoa

- 1 lemon, sliced

- Olive oil

- Salt and pepper

Preparation

- Preheat the oven to 375°F (190°C).

- Place salmon on a baking sheet, arrange asparagus around it, and drizzle with olive oil.

- Add salt and pepper, then bake for 15-20 minutes.

- Serve with quinoa and lemon slices.

Nutritional Information

- Calories: 400

- Protein: 30g

- Carbohydrates: 30g

- Fat: 18g

- Fiber: 6g

Serving Size: 1 serving

Preparation Time: 25 minutes

2. Turkey and Vegetable Stir-Fry

Ingredients

- 6 oz ground turkey

- Mixed stir-fry vegetables (broccoli, bell peppers, snap peas) of 2 Cups

- 1/4 cup diced onion

- 2 cloves garlic, minced

- Low-sodium soy sauce

- Sesame oil (optional)

Preparation

- Cook ground turkey until browned in a skillet.

- Add diced onions and minced garlic, followed by the mixed vegetables.

- Stir-fry until the vegetables are tender.

- Season with low-sodium soy sauce and a drizzle of sesame oil if desired.

Nutritional Information

- Calories: 350

- Protein: 30g

- Carbohydrates: 25g

- Fat: 15g

- Fiber: 6g

Serving Size: 1 serving

Preparation Time: 20 minutes

3. Black Bean Stuffed Bell Peppers and Quinoa

Ingredients

- 2 large bell peppers

- 1 cup cooked quinoa

- Black beans (canned, drained and rinsed) of 1 Cup

- 1/2 cup diced tomatoes

- 1/4 cup diced onions

- 2 tablespoons shredded cheddar cheese (optional)

Preparation

- Preheat the oven to 350°F (175°C).

- Tops of the bell peppers should be cut to remove seeds.

- In a bowl, combine quinoa, black beans, diced tomatoes, and onions.

- Stuff the bell peppers with the quinoa mixture and top with shredded cheese if desired.

- Bake for 25-30 minutes.

Nutritional Information

- Calories: 340

- Protein: 14g

- Carbohydrates: 60g

- Fat: 5g

- Fiber: 12g

Serving Size: 1 stuffed bell pepper

Preparation Time: 40 minutes

4. Spinach and Mushroom Stuffed Chicken Breast

Ingredients

- 6 oz chicken breast

- 1 cup fresh spinach

- 1/4 cup sliced mushrooms

- 2 tablespoons low-fat cream cheese

- Salt and pepper to taste

Preparation

- Preheat the oven to 375°F (190°C).

- Cut a pocket into the chicken breast and stuff with spinach, mushrooms, and cream cheese.

- Season with salt and pepper.

- Bake for 25-30 minutes.

Nutritional Information

- Calories: 330

- Protein: 40g

- Carbohydrates: 6g

- Fat: 16g

- Fiber: 3g

Serving Size: 1 chicken breast

Preparation Time: 35 minutes

5. Lentil and Vegetable Stir-Fry

Ingredients

- Dried green or brown lentils of 1 cup

- 4 cups vegetable broth

- 1 cup diced carrots

- 1 cup diced celery

- 1 cup diced onions

- 2 cloves garlic, minced

- 1 teaspoon cumin

- Salt and pepper to taste

Preparation

- Rinse lentils and combine with vegetable broth in a pot.

- Add vegetables, garlic, cumin, salt, and pepper.

- Simmer for 20-30 minutes until lentils and vegetables are tender.

Nutritional Information

- Calories: 360

- Protein: 20g

- Carbohydrates: 60g

- Fat: 2g

- Fiber: 18g

Serving Size: 1 bowl

Preparation Time: 45 minutes

6. Quinoa and Broccoli Bowl with Tahini Dressing

Ingredients

- 1 cup cooked quinoa

- 1 cup steamed broccoli florets

- 1/4 cup shredded carrots

- 1/4 cup diced red bell peppers

- Tahini dressing

Preparation

- In a bowl, combine quinoa, steamed broccoli, shredded carrots, and diced red bell peppers.

- Drizzle with tahini dressing and toss to combine.

Nutritional Information

- Calories: 340

- Protein: 10g

- Carbohydrates: 45g

- Fat: 15g

- Fiber: 8g

Serving Size: 1 bowl

Preparation Time: 20 minutes

7. Mediterranean Grilled Chicken Salad

Ingredients

- 6 oz grilled chicken breast

- 2 cups mixed greens

- 1/4 cup diced cucumbers

- 1/4 cup cherry tomatoes

- Kalamata olives

- Feta cheese

- Greek dressing

Preparation

- Grill the chicken until cooked through.

- In a bowl, combine mixed greens, cucumbers, and cherry tomatoes.

- Top with grilled chicken, Kalamata olives, and feta cheese.

- Drizzle with Greek dressing.

Nutritional Information

- Calories: 380

- Protein: 40g

- Carbohydrates: 10g

- Fat: 18g

- Fiber: 4g

Serving Size: 1 salad

Preparation Time: 25 minutes

8. Sweet Potato and Chickpea Curry

Ingredients

- 2 cups diced sweet potatoes

- Chickpeas, drained and rinsed of 1 can (15 oz)

- 1/2 cup diced onions

- 1/2 cup diced tomatoes

- 2 cloves garlic, minced

- 1 tablespoon curry powder

- Coconut milk

Preparation

- Sauté onions and garlic until soft in a pot.

- Add diced sweet potatoes and cook for a few minutes.

- Stir in diced tomatoes, chickpeas, and curry powder.

- Add enough water to cover the ingredients and simmer until sweet potatoes are tender.

- Add coconut milk for a creamier texture if desired.

Nutritional Information

- Calories: 340

- Protein: 10g

- Carbohydrates: 60g

- Fat: 8g

- Fiber: 12g

Serving Size: 1 serving

Preparation Time: 35 minutes

9. Spinach and Feta Stuffed Portobello Mushrooms

Ingredients

- 2 large Portobello mushrooms

- 1 cup fresh spinach

- 1/4 cup crumbled feta cheese

- 1 tablespoon olive oil

- Salt and pepper to taste

Preparation

- Preheat the oven to 375°F (190°C).

- Remove the stems from the Portobello mushrooms and brush with olive oil.

- In a pan, sauté fresh spinach until wilted.

- Stuff the mushrooms with sautéed spinach and crumbled feta.

- Season with salt and pepper.

- Bake for 20-25 minutes.

Nutritional Information

- Calories: 320

- Protein: 10g

- Carbohydrates: 10g

- Fat: 25g

- Fiber: 3g

- Serving Size: 1 stuffed mushroom

- Preparation Time: 30 minutes

CHAPTER 4

Snacks Recipes

1. Greek Yogurt Parfait

Ingredients

- 1 cup Greek yogurt

- 1/2 cup mixed berries (strawberries, blueberries, raspberries)

- 1 tablespoon honey

- 1/4 cup granola

Preparation

- Layer Greek yogurt ,mixed berries, honey and granola in a bowl.

- Repeat the layers as desired.

Nutritional Information

- Calories: 250

- Protein: 12g

- Carbohydrates: 35g

- Fat: 8g

- Fiber: 5g

Serving Size: 1 parfait

Preparation Time: 5 minutes

2. Hummus with Veggie Sticks

Ingredients

- 1/4 cup hummus

- Bell pepper strips, Carrot sticks and cucumber slices, and bell pepper strips

Preparation

- Vegetables should be washed and cut into sticks and slices.

- Serve with hummus for dipping.

Nutritional Information

- Calories: 150

- Protein: 5g

- Carbohydrates: 15g

- Fat: 8g

- Fiber: 6g

Serving Size: 1 serving

Preparation Time: 10 minutes

3. Almond Butter and Banana Rice Cakes

Ingredients

- 2 rice cakes
- 2 tablespoons almond butter
- 1 ripe banana, sliced

Preparation

- Spread almond butter on rice cakes.
- Top with sliced bananas.

Nutritional Information

- Calories: 300
- Protein: 7g
- Carbohydrates: 40g
- Fat: 14g
- Fiber: 6g

Serving Size: 2 rice cakes

Preparation Time: 5 minutes

4. Trail Mix

Ingredients

- 1/4 cup almonds

- 1/4 cup walnuts

- 1/4 cup dried cranberries

- 1/4 cup dark chocolate chips

Preparation

- Mix all ingredients in a bowl.

- Portion into snack-sized bags for easy grab-and-go.

Nutritional Information

- Calories: 300

- Protein: 7g

- Carbohydrates: 25g

- Fat: 20g

- Fiber: 4g

Serving Size: 1/4 cup mix

Preparation Time: 5 minutes

5. Cottage Cheese and Pineapple

Ingredients

- 1/2 cup low-fat cottage cheese

- 1/2 cup diced fresh pineapple

Preparation

- Place cottage cheese in a bowl and top with diced pineapple.

Nutritional Information

- Calories: 150

- Protein: 15g

- Carbohydrates: 18g

- Fat: 2g

- Fiber: 2g

Serving Size: 1 serving

Preparation Time: 5 minutes

6. Apple Slices with Almond Butter

Ingredients

- 1 apple, sliced

- 2 tablespoons almond butter

Preparation

- Slice the apple into rounds or wedges.

- Dip in almond butter for a delicious snack.

Nutritional Information

- Calories: 250

- Protein: 6g

- Carbohydrates: 25g

- Fat: 16g

- Fiber: 6g

Serving Size: 1 serving

Preparation Time: 5 minutes

7. Caprese Skewers

Ingredients

- Cherry tomatoes

- Fresh basil leaves

- Mozzarella balls

- Balsamic glaze for drizzling

Preparation

- Thread cherry tomatoes, basil leaves, and mozzarella balls onto skewers.

- Drizzle with balsamic glaze.

Nutritional Information

- Calories: 180

- Protein: 10g

- Carbohydrates: 5g

- Fat: 12g

- Fiber: 1g

Serving Size: 2 skewers

Preparation Time: 10 minutes

8. Tuna Salad Lettuce Wraps

Ingredients

- 1 can (5 oz) tuna, drained

- 2 tablespoons Greek yogurt

- 1/4 cup diced celery

- 1/4 cup diced red onion

- Lettuce leaves for wrapping

Preparation

- In a bowl, mix tuna, Greek yogurt, celery, and red onion.

- Spoon the tuna salad into lettuce leaves and wrap them up.

Nutritional Information

- Calories: 200

- Protein: 20g

- Carbohydrates: 6g

- Fat: 10g

- Fiber: 1g

Serving Size: 1 serving

Preparation Time: 10 minutes

9. Popcorn with Nutritional Yeast

Ingredients

- Air-popped popcorn
- 2 tablespoons nutritional yeast
- Any seasonings you desire (e.g., paprika, garlic powder)

Preparation

- Pop the popcorn using an air popper.
- Sprinkle nutritional yeast and seasonings for added flavor.

Nutritional Information

- Calories: 100
- Protein: 3g
- Carbohydrates: 20g
- Fat: 1g
- Fiber: 4g

Serving Size: 2 cups

Preparation Time: 5 minutes

10. Cucumber and Dill Greek Yogurt Dip

Ingredients

- 1 cup Greek yogurt

- 1 cucumber, finely grated and drained

- 1 clove garlic, minced

- 2 tablespoons fresh dill, chopped

- Salt and pepper to taste

Preparation

- In a bowl, combine Greek yogurt, grated cucumber, garlic, and dill.

- Season with salt and pepper.

- Serve with fresh vegetable sticks or whole-grain crackers.

Nutritional Information

- Calories: 120

- Protein: 10g

- Carbohydrates: 10g

- Fat: 4g

- Fiber: 1g

- Serving Size: 2 tablespoons

- Preparation Time: 10 minutes

CHAPTER 5

7 DAYS MEAL PLAN

Day 1

- **Breakfast:** Berry and Greek Yogurt Parfait

- **Lunch:** Grilled Chicken and Quinoa Salad

- **Dinner:** Spinach and Feta Stuffed Portobello Mushrooms

Day 2

- **Breakfast:** Avocado and Spinach Breakfast Wrap

- **Lunch:** Lentil and Vegetable Soup

- **Dinner:** Turkey and Vegetable Stir-Fry

Day 3

- **Breakfast**: Oatmeal with Almonds and Banana

- **Lunch**: Quinoa and Black Bean Salad

- **Dinner**: Spinach and Mushroom Stuffed Chicken Breast

Day 4

- **Breakfast**: Vegetable and Goat Cheese Omelet

- **Lunch**: Chickpea and Spinach Salad

- **Dinner:** Sweet Potato and Chickpea Curry

Day 5

- **Breakfast**: Smoothie Bowl with Spinach and Berries

- **Lunch**: Tuna and White Bean Salad

- **Dinner**: Lentil and Vegetable Stir-Fry

Day 6

- **Breakfast:** Quinoa Breakfast Bowl

- **Lunch**: Quinoa and Black Bean Salad

- **Dinner:** Quinoa and Broccoli Bowl with Tahini Dressing

Day 7

- **Breakfast:** Chia Seed Pudding with Mango

- **Lunch**: Black Bean Salsa with Baked Sweet Potato

- **Dinner**: Mediterranean Grilled Chicken Salad

CHAPTER 6

CONCLUSION

Anyone wishing to maintain their health and well-being while living with multiple sclerosis will find the "Overcoming Multiple Sclerosis Diet Cookbook for Seniors" to be an invaluable resource. We've looked through a number of delectable and nourishing recipes on these pages that are intended to help people with MS on their path to better health and a higher standard of living.

Although having multiple sclerosis might be difficult, it also presents a chance to adopt a healthy lifestyle and make wise decisions. With the help of this cookbook, people with MS of all ages may now take control of their nutrition, try new foods, and make educated food choices.

We now know that food can be an effective ally in the battle against MS symptoms, and these dishes demonstrate that eating well doesn't have to compromise flavor or appeal.

We commend all of the elderly and MS patients who have started this culinary adventure for their dedication to their health and wellbeing. There are many obstacles on the road to beating multiple sclerosis, but there are also plenty of delectable, healthy, and fulfilling meals along the way. I hope that this cookbook will be a constant source of motivation and strength for you as you pursue a happy, full life.

We are appreciative that you have selected the "Overcoming Multiple Sclerosis Diet Cookbook for Seniors" as your reference. The kitchen will always be your canvas for a thriving, healthy future as you continue your journey.

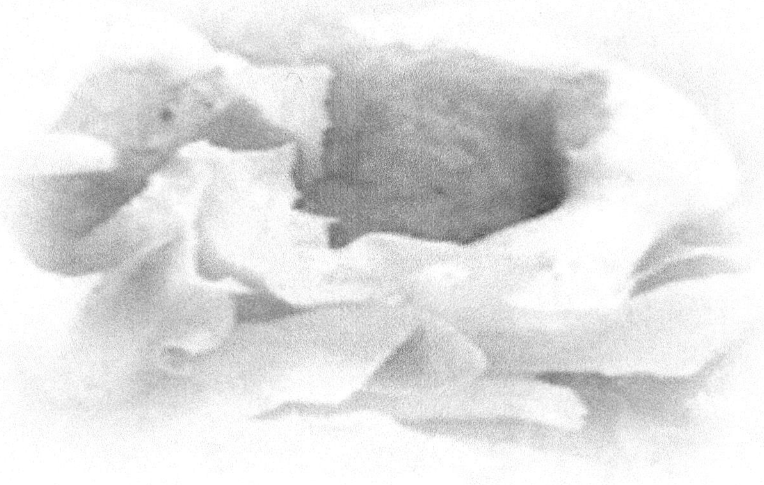

THANKS FOR READING